Stroke

Signs, Symptoms, Causes, Types and Prevention

Dr. Sheila Harrison

Disclaimer

This content serves to provide general information about the disease and aims to empower you to seek prompt medical assistance if necessary to prevent complications. It's essential to stress that this information is not a substitute for consulting a qualified physician. The field of medical science is continually evolving, and due to the dynamic nature of medical knowledge, we recommend seeking expert advice if you encounter any inconsistencies or intend to take action based on the information in this content. Never disregard professional medical guidance or delay treatment based on something you've read online, including this material, or from any other online source. Always remember that the internet cannot cure you; rather, healing comes through the guidance of medical professionals and the providence of God.

Table of Content

Review

A stroke is like a heart attack for your brain, and it's a serious, life-threatening emergency. Quick action is crucial because delays in care can lead to lasting brain damage or even death. Strokes can be scary for those going through them or those around them.

Fortunately, there are more and better treatment options for strokes now. Advances in understanding the brain, improved imaging technology, and new medications contribute to this progress. If you notice stroke symptoms in yourself or someone else, getting immediate medical attention is vital. The sooner a person having a stroke receives care, the more likely the effects can be limited or reversed.

Swift treatment can make a significant difference, turning a potentially disabling or deadly event into something more manageable. Knowing how to recognize stroke signs and taking the right actions can save a life and reduce complications. Lifestyle changes can also help lower the risk of stroke. Explore more about the types, early signs, symptoms, causes of stroke, and discover ways to prevent it.

Who does Stroke affect?

Strokes can affect anyone, whether they're children or adults, but certain individuals face a higher risk. Strokes are more prevalent in older age, with about two-thirds occurring in people over 65.

Certain medical conditions can elevate the risk of stroke. These include high blood pressure (hypertension), high cholesterol (hyperlipidemia), Type 2 diabetes, and individuals with a history of stroke, heart attack, or irregular heart rhythms like atrial fibrillation.

How common is a stroke?

Strokes are widespread, ranking as the second leading cause of death globally. In the United States, they hold the position of the fifth leading cause of death. Additionally, strokes are a major contributor to disability on a global scale.

Section 1

What is stroke?

A stroke is a critical condition that occurs when a portion of your brain lacks sufficient blood flow. This typically results from either a blocked artery or bleeding within the brain. When the affected area doesn't receive a consistent blood supply, the brain cells in that region begin to die due to a shortage of oxygen.

or

A stroke happens when the blood supply to certain parts of the brain is diminished or interrupted. This leads to a deprivation of essential nutrients and oxygen required for the survival of brain tissue. Within a matter of minutes, cells begin to die, adversely affecting brain functions.

URGENT: A stroke is a critical emergency, and time is of the essence. If you or someone around you displays symptoms of a stroke, CALL 911 (or your local emergency services number) IMMEDIATELY. Swift treatment significantly increases the likelihood of recovery without lasting disability.A person experiencing a stroke may have muscle weakness on one side. Request them to raise their arms. If there's one-sided weakness (newly occurring), one arm will stay higher while the other sags and drops.

To identify the warning signs of a stroke, remember the acronym **BE FAST**:

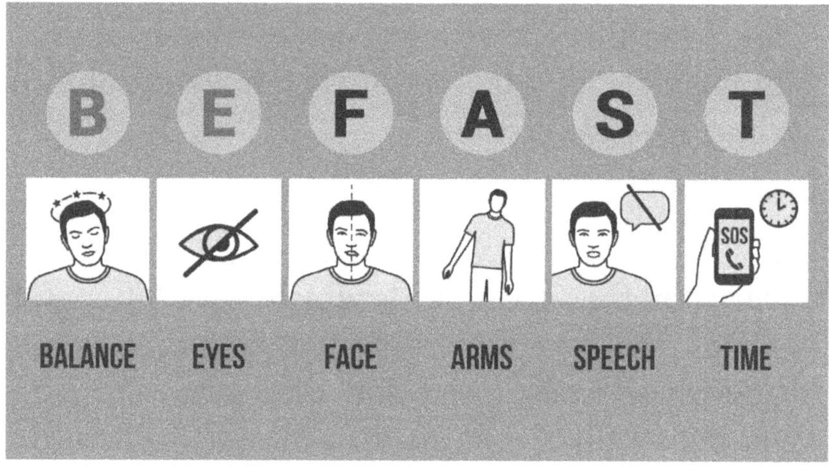

- **B**: Be watchful for a sudden loss of balance.
- **E**: Look out for a sudden loss of vision in one or both eyes. Check for double vision
- **F**: Ask the person to smile. Observe for a droop on one or both sides of their face, indicating muscle weakness or paralysis..
- **A**: A person having a stroke often has muscle weakness on one side. Ask them to raise their arms. If they have one-sided weakness (and

didn't have it before), one arm will stay higher while the other will sag and drop downward.

- **S**: Strokes can affect a person's ability to speak. Watch for slurred speech or difficulty choosing the right words.
- **T**: Time is crucial, so don't delay in seeking help! If possible, check the time symptoms begin. Informing a healthcare provider about the onset of symptoms helps them determine the most appropriate treatment options

How does a stroke affect my body?

Strokes are akin to heart attacks for your brain. During a stroke, a section of your brain loses its blood supply, depriving it of oxygen. Without oxygen, the affected brain cells become oxygen-starved and cease to function correctly.

If the brain cells remain without oxygen for an extended period, they will die. When a sufficient number of brain cells in an area die, the damage becomes irreversible, leading to the potential loss of abilities controlled by that region. However, restoring blood flow can prevent or at least limit such damage. This underscores the critical importance of time in the treatment of a stroke.

Section 2

Types of Stroke

Strokes can occur through two primary mechanisms: ischemia and hemorrhage.

Ischemic stroke

Ischemia (pronounced "iss-key-me-uh") occurs when cells do not receive sufficient blood flow to provide them with oxygen. This commonly happens due to an obstruction in the blood vessels of your brain, leading to a cutoff in blood flow. Ischemic strokes are the most prevalent, constituting approximately 80% of all strokes.

Ischemic strokes typically occur through one of the following mechanisms:

- Formation of a clot in your brain (thrombosis).
- A fragment of a clot that originated elsewhere in your body breaks free and travels through your blood vessels until it becomes lodged in your brain (embolism).
- Small vessel blockage (lacunar stroke), which may result from untreated, long-term high blood pressure (hypertension), high

cholesterol (hyperlipidemia), or high blood sugar (Type 2 diabetes).high cholesterol (hyperlipidemia) or high blood sugar (Type 2 diabetes).

- Unknown reasons (referred to as cryptogenic strokes; "cryptogenic" means "hidden origin").

Hemorrhagic stroke

Hemorrhagic (pronounced "hem-or-aj-ick") strokes result in bleeding in or around your brain, occurring in one of two ways:

- Bleeding inside your brain (intracerebral): This happens when a blood vessel inside your brain tears or ruptures, leading to bleeding that exerts pressure on the surrounding brain tissue.

- Bleeding into the subarachnoid space (the space between your brain and its outer covering): The arachnoid membrane, a thin tissue layer with a spiderweb-like pattern, surrounds your brain. The area between it and your brain is the subarachnoid space ("sub" means "under"). Damage to blood vessels passing through the arachnoid membrane can cause a subarachnoid hemorrhage, involving bleeding into the subarachnoid space and exerting pressure on the underlying brain tissue.

Section 3

Symptoms of Stroke

A simple way to remember stroke symptoms is the word FAST, emphasizing the importance of swift treatment:

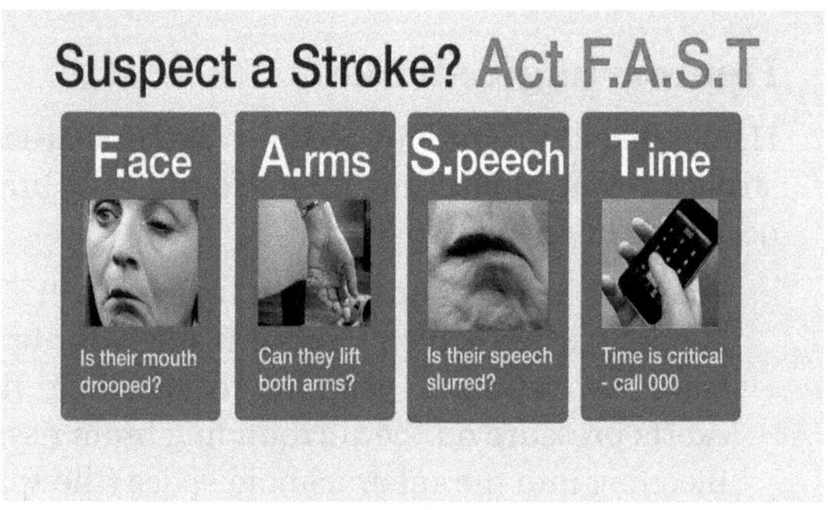

- **F** is for face droop,
- **A** is for uneven arm weakness,
- **S** is for speech problems, and
- **T** is for time. Quick care is crucial.

Stroke symptoms vary depending on the affected area of the brain, as different regions control different abilities. For instance, a stroke impacting Broca's area, responsible for controlling facial and mouth muscles used in speech, may lead to slurred speech or difficulty speaking.

Symptoms of a stroke may involve one or more of the following:

- One-sided weakness or paralysis.
- Aphasia (difficulty with or loss of speaking ability).
- Slurred or garbled speaking (dysarthria).
- Loss of muscle control on one side of your face.
- Sudden loss — either partial or total — of one or more senses (vision, hearing, smell, taste and touch).
- Blurred or double vision (diplopia).
- Loss of coordination or clumsiness (ataxia).
- Dizziness or vertigo.
- Nausea and vomiting.
- Neck stiffness.
- Emotional instability and personality changes.
- Confusion or agitation.
- Seizures.
- Memory loss (amnesia).
- Headaches (usually sudden and severe).
- Passing out or fainting.
- Coma.

Transient ischemic attack (TIA)

A transient ischemic attack (TIA), sometimes referred to as a "mini-stroke," resembles a stroke, but its effects are temporary. TIAs often serve as warning signs that an individual has a significantly elevated risk of experiencing a full-fledged stroke in the near future. Consequently, immediate emergency medical care is essential for someone who has had a TIA.

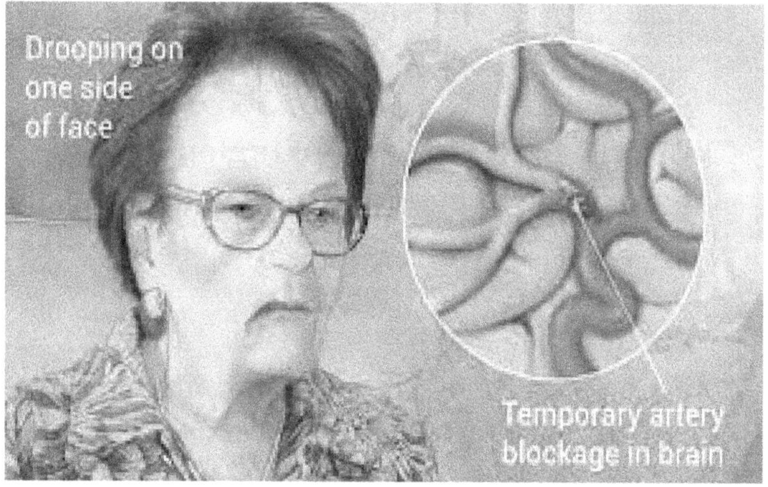

Section 4
Causes Of stroke

Ischemic strokes and hemorrhagic strokes can occur for various reasons. Ischemic strokes typically result from blood clots, and these clots can form due to a range of factors, including:

- **Atherosclerosis:** A condition where fatty deposits (plaque) build up in your arteries, narrowing and potentially blocking blood flow.
- **Clotting disorders:** Conditions that affect the normal clotting of blood, making it more prone to forming clots, which can lead to blockages in blood vessels.
- **Atrial fibrillation:** An irregular heart rhythm that can lead to the formation of blood clots in the heart, increasing the risk of strokes.
- **Heart defects (atrial septal defect or ventricular septal defect):** Structural abnormalities in the heart that can create conditions favoring the formation of blood clots, potentially causing strokes.
- **Microvascular ischemic disease:** Small blood vessels in the brain can be affected, leading to reduced blood flow and an increased risk of stroke.

Hemorrhagic strokes may occur due to various reasons, including:

- **High blood pressure:** Particularly when it persists over an extended period, reaches very high levels, or both.
- **Brain aneurysms:** Certain cases of these bulging blood vessel weak points can result in hemorrhagic strokes.
- **Brain tumors:** Including cancerous growths in the brain.
- **Diseases affecting blood vessels in the brain:** Conditions like moyamoya disease that weaken or bring about abnormal changes in brain blood vessels.

Related conditions

Various other conditions and factors can contribute to an individual's risk of experiencing a stroke. These encompass:

- Alcohol use disorder.
- High blood pressure: It plays a role in all types of strokes by contributing to blood vessel damage, increasing the likelihood of a stroke.
- High cholesterol (hyperlipidemia).

- Migraine headaches: Especially those with auras, as they can exhibit symptoms similar to a stroke, and individuals with migraines have an elevated risk of stroke at some point in their lives.
- Type 2 diabetes.
- Smoking and other forms of tobacco use: This includes vaping and smokeless tobacco.
- Drug misuse: Involving both prescription and non-prescription drugs.

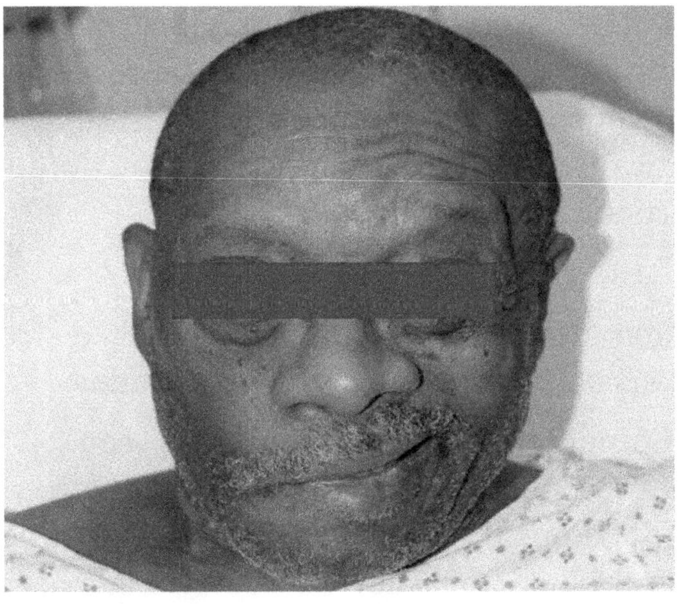

Is it contagious?

Strokes aren't contagious and you can't pass them to or get them from other people.

Section 5
Diagnosis and Tests

Stroke Diagnosis

A healthcare professional can identify a stroke through a comprehensive process involving a neurological examination, diagnostic imaging, and additional tests. In the neurological examination, you'll be asked to perform specific tasks or answer questions. While you engage in these activities, the provider will observe for distinctive signs indicating an issue with the functioning of a particular part of your brain.

When a healthcare provider suspects a stroke, the most common tests conducted include:

- Computerized tomography (CT) scan.
- Lab blood tests: These assess for signs of infections or heart damage, check clotting ability and blood sugar levels, and evaluate kidney and liver function, among other factors.
- Electrocardiogram (ECG or EKG): Ensures that a heart issue is not the underlying cause.
- Magnetic resonance imaging (MRI) scans.

- Electroencephalogram (EEG): Although less common, it can rule out seizures or related problems.

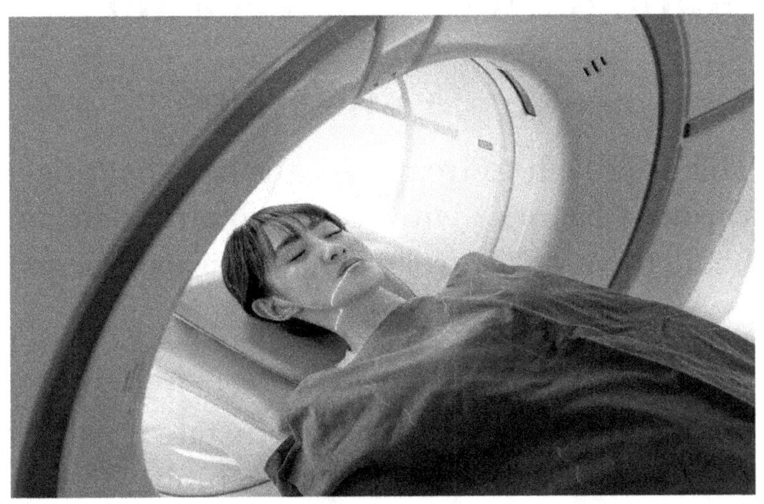

Computerized tomography (CT) scan

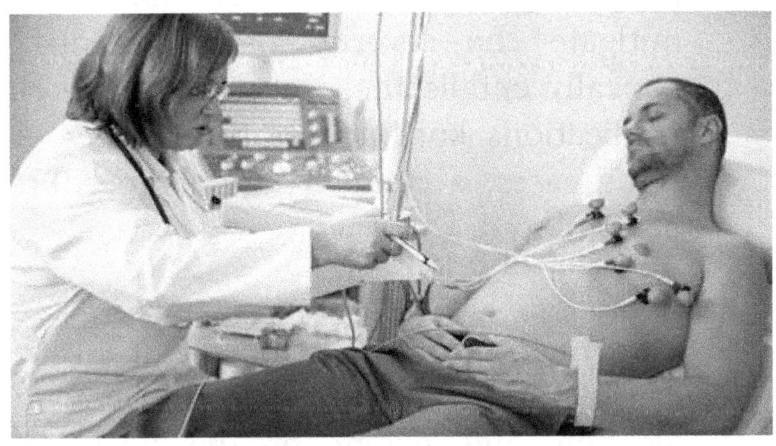

Electrocardiogram (ECG or EKG)

Section 6

Management and Treatment

How are strokes treated?

The approach to treating a stroke is contingent on various factors, with the primary determinant being the type of stroke a person is experiencing.

- **Ischemic:** In the case of ischemic strokes, the foremost objective is to reinstate circulation to the impacted areas of the brain. If achieved promptly, it is sometimes feasible to avert permanent damage or, at the very least, mitigate the severity of the stroke. This typically entails the use of a specific class of medications known as thrombolytics, and in some cases, a catheterization procedure may be employed.

- **Hemorrhagic:** For hemorrhagic strokes, the course of treatment is contingent on the location and extent of the bleeding. The primary focus is often on lowering blood pressure, as this can diminish the amount of bleeding and prevent its escalation. Enhancing clotting to halt the bleeding is another treatment avenue. In certain instances, surgery may be required to alleviate pressure on the brain caused by accumulated blood.

What medications or treatments are used?

The medications and treatments administered depend on the type of stroke and the timeliness of treatment initiation after the event. Long-term treatments for stroke are implemented in the days and months following emergency intervention that addresses the immediate threat of a stroke.

In essence, your healthcare provider is the most qualified individual to advise on the recommended treatment(s). They can customize the information to your specific case, considering factors such as your medical history, personal circumstances, and more.

Some examples of treatments for stroke are as follows:

Ischemic stroke	Hemorrhagic stroke
Thrombolytic drugs (within three to four and a half hours).	Blood pressure management.
Thrombectomy (within 24 hours if there's no significant brain damage).	Reversal of any medication that might increase bleeding.
Blood pressure management.	Use of medications or surgery to reduce pressure inside your skull.

Thrombolytic drugs

Thrombolytic drugs, derived from the Greek words "thrombus" meaning "clot" and "lysis" meaning "loosening/dissolving," are a viable option within the initial three hours after the onset of stroke symptoms. These medications are designed to dissolve existing blood clots. However, their effectiveness is limited to the three- to four-and-a-half hour window because beyond that timeframe, they raise the risk of potentially hazardous bleeding complications.

Mechanical thrombectomy

In situations where thrombolytic drugs are not a viable option, particularly when time has elapsed, a catheterization procedure called mechanical thrombectomy becomes a potential alternative. Mechanical thrombectomy procedures also have a time-sensitive nature, with the optimal window being within 24 hours of symptom onset. This procedure entails inserting a catheter (tube-like device) into a major blood vessel and navigating it to the clot in the brain. At the clot site, the catheter is equipped with a tool at its tip designed to extract the clot.

Blood pressure management

Since elevated blood pressure is often the cause of hemorrhagic strokes, a crucial aspect of their treatment involves reducing blood pressure. Lowering blood pressure plays a pivotal role in restricting bleeding and facilitates the clotting process to seal the damaged blood vessel.

Clotting support

The body's clotting ability, essential for stopping bleeding and healing injuries, depends on a process known as hemostasis. To aid hemostasis, medications or blood factors are administered to facilitate clotting. Examples include vitamin K therapy, infusions of prothrombin or clotting factors, among others. This form of treatment is predominantly employed in cases of hemorrhagic strokes and proves beneficial in controlling bleeding, particularly for individuals on blood-thinning medications.

Surgery

In certain situations, surgery becomes imperative to alleviate pressure on the brain. This necessity is particularly pronounced in cases of subarachnoid hemorrhages, which are more accessible as they occur on the outer surface of the brain.

Supportive treatments and other methods

Stroke treatment encompasses various approaches, some directly supportive and others focused on preventing complications. Specific details about these additional treatments, along with recommendations and explanations, can be provided by your healthcare provider.

Stroke rehabilitation

An integral aspect of stroke treatment involves aiding individuals in their recovery or adaptation to the changes in their brain, particularly in helping them regain lost abilities. Stroke rehabilitation plays a crucial role in the recovery process for most individuals who have experienced a stroke. This rehabilitation can assume various forms, encompassing:

- **Speech therapy:** This assists in recovering language and speaking abilities, enhancing control over muscles involved in breathing, eating, drinking, and swallowing.
- **Physical therapy:** Aimed at improving or restoring the use of hands, arms, feet, and legs, as well as addressing balance issues, muscle weakness, and related concerns.

- **Occupational therapy:** Focuses on retraining the brain to facilitate everyday activities, with a particular emphasis on refining fine motor skills and muscle control.
- **Cognitive therapy:** Beneficial for addressing memory issues and difficulties with activities requiring focus or concentration that may have been previously manageable.

Additional therapies may be considered based on your individual case and needs. Your healthcare provider is the most qualified person to provide guidance on which treatments would be most beneficial for you.

How soon after treatment will I feel better?

The duration of recovery and the time it takes to experience improvement after treatment vary based on several factors. Your healthcare provider is the most reliable source to provide information on what to expect and the probable timeline for your recovery.

Section 7

Complications/side effects of the treatment

The potential side effects of stroke treatments are highly dependent on factors such as the type of stroke, the specific treatments employed, and individual medical history. Your healthcare provider is the best resource to provide information on the expected side effects and guidance on how to manage or prevent them.

How can I take care of myself or manage the symptoms?

It's important to note that a stroke is a critical medical emergency, and attempting to self-diagnose or self-treat is not recommended. If you or someone around you is experiencing stroke symptoms, immediate action is crucial. Call 911 (or your local emergency services number) promptly, as delaying stroke treatment increases the risk of permanent brain damage or fatality.

A stroke is a critical and life-threatening medical emergency, and attempting self-diagnosis or self-treatment is strongly discouraged. If you or someone with you exhibits symptoms of a stroke, it is imperative to call 911 (or your local emergency services number) immediately. Swift initiation of stroke treatment is essential, as any delay increases the risk of permanent brain damage or even death.

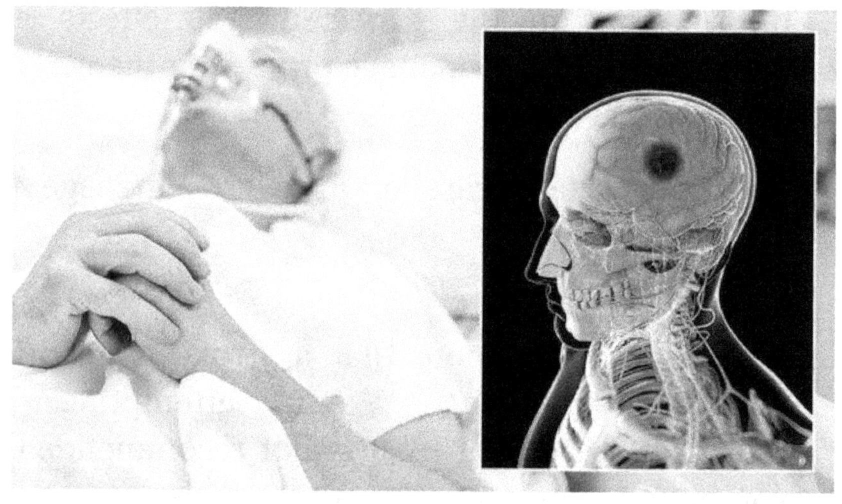

Stroke Paient on a life support

Scetion 8

How do I take care of myself Living With Stroke

In the event of a stroke, your healthcare provider will collaborate with you to devise a treatment plan and outline the anticipated timeline for recovery. They may prescribe medications, suggest therapy options, and more. It is crucial to engage in a conversation with your healthcare provider to understand the rationale behind their recommendations and how these measures can benefit you.

Following the finalized treatment plan diligently is of utmost importance as it offers the best opportunity to optimize your recovery. Additionally, consider the following steps:

- **Adherence to Medication:** Take prescribed medications consistently, as they can play a crucial role in preventing another stroke.

- **Attendance of Rehabilitation/Therapy Appointments:** Regular attendance and active participation in rehabilitation or therapy sessions are vital for your recovery.

- **Prioritize Mental Health:** Depression and anxiety are common after a stroke. Seeking help for these conditions is important, as untreated mental health issues can hinder the recovery process. Discuss any such feelings with your healthcare provider to explore appropriate care.

- **Implement Lifestyle Changes:** Make an effort to adopt recommended lifestyle changes, especially regarding blood pressure, blood sugar, and cholesterol management. Addressing these factors can contribute significantly to both your recovery and preventing future strokes. If you use tobacco or vaping products, quitting can also have substantial benefits..

Section 9

Prevention of Stroke

Certain risk factors for stroke, like age and family history, are beyond our control. However, adopting specific lifestyle habits can substantially diminish the risk of experiencing a stroke. While these measures do not guarantee stroke prevention, they contribute to lowering the overall risk. Here are actions you can take:

- **Improve Lifestyle:** Improve your lifestyle: Eating a healthy diet and adding exercise to your daily routine can improve your health. You should also make sure to get enough sleep (the recommended amount is seven to eight hours).

- **Lower your blood pressure:** High blood pressure is one of the top causes of stroke. However, we may not always know that we have hypertension since it often does not show any symptoms. Hence, for those with normal blood pressure levels, it is recommended that we take a blood pressure reading at least once every 3 years.

- **Avoid smoking:** It is commonly known that smoking is harmful to our bodies, including raising our risk of stroke. If you don't smoke, don't start. If you do smoke, get support, and quit smoking today to reduce your stroke risk.

- **Take note of your heart health:** If you have pre-existing heart conditions, make sure you consult your doctor and follow their advice to keep it under control, to reduce your risk of stroke.

- **Stay active:** Exercising can help us lose weight and reduce the likelihood of us developing health conditions such as diabetes, hypertension, and high cholesterol, which are risk factors of stroke. You can start small by choosing to take the stairs instead of the escalator and taking the longer route home. Doing a short 30-minutes workout at home, 5 days a week, can also help.

- **Limit your alcohol intake:** Drink in moderation, or not at all. To prevent any health complications caused by excessive alcohol intake, ladies should limit themselves to 1 drink a day, while men should only have up to 2 drinks a day.

- **Adopt a healthy diet:** Load up on fresh fruits and vegetables and cut down your intake of salt and trans and saturated fats, which can clog our arteries and raise blood pressure. Eating healthy can also help us shed some weight, further reducing our stroke risk.

- **Manage your diabetes:** If you have diabetes, keep it under control with regular exercise, a healthy diet, and medication prescribed by your doctor.

- **Watch your cholesterol levels:** Exercising regularly and sticking to a healthy diet can help to reduce your cholesterol levels, but sometimes it may not be enough. Sometimes, doctors may prescribe medication to help keep your cholesterol in check.

- **Take your medication:** For those with an existing health condition that raises your risk of stroke, make sure you follow your doctor's advice and keep it under control. If you have had a stroke previously, make sure to take any medication your doctor prescribes to prevent another one.

See your primary care provider for a checkup or wellness visit annually. Yearly wellness visits can detect health problems — especially ones that contribute to having a stroke — long before you feel any symptoms.

NOTE: Stroke recovery is a gradual process that can take several months to years. Besides professional medical care and rehabilitation therapy, familial support can go a long way in helping your loved ones regain independence and rediscover self-confidence.

Find out how you can make a difference to your loved one's recovery post-stroke by connecting with support groups.

Stroke Prevention Summary

Make informed decisions about your lifestyle to minimize risks or alter behaviors that could jeopardize your health. Specific practices, such as smoking, tobacco use (including vaping), recreational drug use, prescription drug misuse, and excessive alcohol consumption, can heighten the likelihood of experiencing a stroke. It is crucial to either cease these behaviors or refrain from starting them altogether. If you encounter challenges in overcoming these habits, consult with your healthcare provider. They can provide guidance and access to resources that support lifestyle changes.

Effectively manage your health conditions and risk factors. Certain conditions, including obesity, abnormal heart rhythms, sleep apnea, high blood pressure, Type 2 diabetes, or high cholesterol, elevate the risk of ischemic stroke. If you have one or more of these conditions, proactive management is vital. Follow your healthcare provider's recommendations, especially regarding medications such as blood thinners, to mitigate the risk of severe stroke-related complications later in life.

Section 10

First Aid to a New Stroke Patient

Immediate actions are crucial when a stroke occurs, aiming to minimize potential brain damage. Here are the recommended first aid steps for a new stroke patient:

Call 911 Immediately:

Time is critical in stroke treatment, as brain cells perish with each passing minute.

If someone exhibits stroke symptoms, dial 911 rather than attempting to transport them to the hospital yourself.

This ensures swift transportation, and paramedics can identify symptoms, provide life-saving treatment, and inform the emergency department.

Take Note of Symptom Onset Time:

Effective stroke treatments must be administered within 6 hours of symptom onset.

Being aware of when the symptoms began helps determine the most appropriate and timely treatment.

Perform CPR if Necessary:

In some cases, a person may lose consciousness during a stroke.

If consciousness is lost, check pulse and breathing; if absent, commence CPR immediately.

Avoid Food or Drink:

Refrain from offering food or drink during a suspected stroke, considering the risk of swallowing difficulty due to muscle weakness or paralysis.

Do Not Administer Medication:

Different strokes may require distinct treatments; for instance, aspirin might help with an ischemic stroke but could be harmful in a hemorrhagic stroke.

Without knowledge of the stroke type, it's advisable not to administer medication to prevent potential complications.

Post-stroke Care:

Understanding how to recognize stroke signs and take immediate action is essential. The next phase involves aiding your loved one in post-stroke recovery, which is a gradual process spanning months to years. Familial support plays a crucial role in helping them regain independence and rebuild self-confidence.

Section 11

Dysphagia after Stroke: Things You Should Know

According to studies, dysphagia affects 50% of acute stroke patients. If untreated, it could lead to serious health complications and even death.

What is Dysphagia?

Dysphagia is a medical term that refers to difficulty or discomfort in swallowing. It can occur at different stages of the swallowing process, including the oral phase (chewing and forming a bolus), the pharyngeal phase (initiating the swallow reflex), and the esophageal phase (moving the bolus into the stomach). Dysphagia can be a result of various medical conditions, including neurological disorders, muscular disorders, structural abnormalities, or other underlying health issues.

Symptoms of dysphagia may include:

- Difficulty initiating a swallow

- Choking or coughing during or after eating or drinking
- Feeling of food sticking in the throat or chest
- Regurgitation of food
- Unintended weight loss
- Recurrent pneumonia or respiratory issues due to food entering the airway
- Avoidance of certain foods or liquids

The causes of dysphagia can vary, ranging from conditions like stroke, Parkinson's disease, or muscular dystrophy to structural issues such as tumors or strictures in the esophagus. It's crucial to consult with a healthcare professional if someone is experiencing symptoms of dysphagia, as proper diagnosis and management are essential for effective treatment and to prevent complications like malnutrition or aspiration pneumonia. Treatment approaches may involve dietary modifications, swallowing exercises, and, in some cases, medical interventions or surgery.

If you or your loved one is recovering from a stroke, you'll need to be careful with swallowing issues. In medical terms, this is known as dysphagia. Those with dysphagia will have difficulties swallowing certain foods or liquids; in more severe cases, some people are unable to do so.

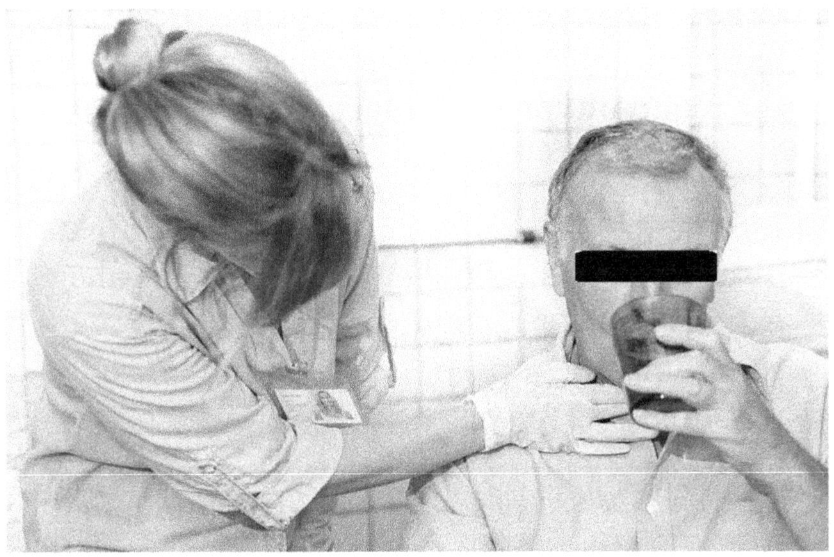

Swallowing is a complex process that involves the coordinated effort of numerous muscles and nerves. When we chew food, it forms a soft ball, known as a bolus, that is prepared for swallowing. The act of swallowing triggers a sequence of movements in the mouth and throat, ensuring that the entrance to the windpipe is covered, allowing the bolus to enter the esophagus—a tube that transports food and liquids to the stomach.

During swallowing, peristalsis—a natural wave-like movement—propels the bolus through the esophagus and into the stomach. At the junction of the esophagus and stomach, there is a muscular band that should open to permit the passage of food into the stomach and close tightly to prevent the regurgitation of stomach acid.

Dysphagia, a condition marked by difficulty or discomfort in swallowing, can lead to challenges in eating, drinking, and proper swallowing. This condition may pose health risks, such as the possibility of aspiration, where food or drink enters the windpipe instead of the esophagus, or an inability to move food or drink down into the stomach. Understanding dysphagia is essential for individuals and their loved ones to navigate recovery effectively.

Stroke and Dysphagia

A stroke occurs when the blood supply to parts of the brain is either reduced or interrupted, leading to impaired blood flow and the potential for brain damage, which may result in disability. There are two main types of strokes: ischemic, caused by a blood vessel blockage, and hemorrhagic, resulting from a blood vessel leak or rupture.

The aftermath of a stroke can significantly impact the ability to chew and swallow, giving rise to various complications:

- If the stroke affects the arms, it may be challenging to use cutlery or grasp items.

- Facial muscle impairment can hinder mouth movement and lead to drooling.

- Balance issues stemming from the stroke can affect swallowing.

Aspiration, the inhalation of food, drink, or saliva into the lungs, is a common complication. Stroke-induced reduction in sensation may result in silent aspiration, where individuals may not be aware of inhaling substances into the lungs.

Who is At Risk?

Anyone recovering from a stroke is at risk of having dysphagia, but elderly persons fall in the higher risk category. In some cases, some people may recover quickly after a stroke, either due to early intervention when the stroke first occurred or due to other circumstances (e.g., responding well to treatment).In many instances, individuals may experience a swift recovery after a stroke, attributed to prompt intervention during the initial occurrence or favorable responses to treatment. Despite such positive outcomes, the risk of developing dysphagia remains heightened, particularly for elderly individuals. The recovery process, especially for seniors, often extends beyond conventional timelines. Caregivers may find themselves taking an active role in feeding their loved ones, as lingering challenges could persist even after substantial mobility improvement. Vigilant monitoring becomes imperative to avert potential dysphagia-related complications. Additionally, ongoing follow-up checks and tailored treatments may be essential for a comprehensive recovery.

The recovery journey from a stroke is often protracted, particularly for elderly individuals. It may necessitate an extended duration compared to typical recovery periods. Caregivers may find themselves actively involved in the feeding process, especially if their loved ones encounter challenges in self-care. Despite significant strides in mobility recovery, ongoing vigilance is crucial. Frequent monitoring remains imperative to forestall potential complications related to dysphagia, ensuring a comprehensive and sustained rehabilitation process.

Follow-up checks and treatment may be needed to help you or your loved one to make a full recovery.

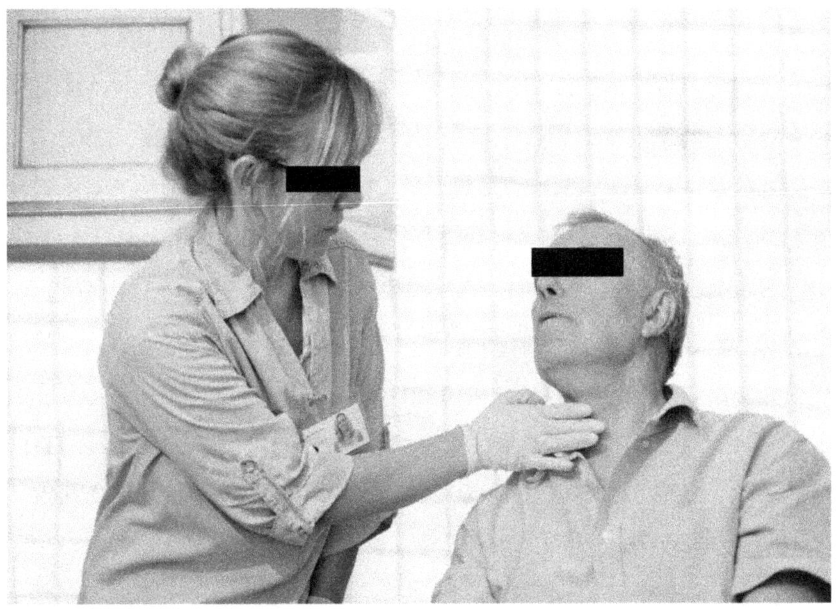

Frequent monitoring

When Can Dysphagia Occur?

Dysphagia can occur during any of the three main phases of swallowing.

- **Oral:** this pertains to the mouth, or when food is being chewed up into a bolus before it's moved to the esophagus. Complications may affect the tongue or even the muscles that allow you to chew food

- **Oropharyngeal:** this pertains to the throat; a stroke can potentially weaken the throat muscles, which thus complicates the swallowing process. You or your loved one could potentially choke, gag, or cough; the food or drink could also go down the windpipe and cause (silent) aspiration

- **Oesophageal:** this pertains to the esophagus; it could refer to food that gets caught or stuck at the base of your throat or in your chest once you've started to swallow

Whenever dysphagia occurs at any stage, seek immediate medical attention.

Signs and Symptoms of Dysphagia

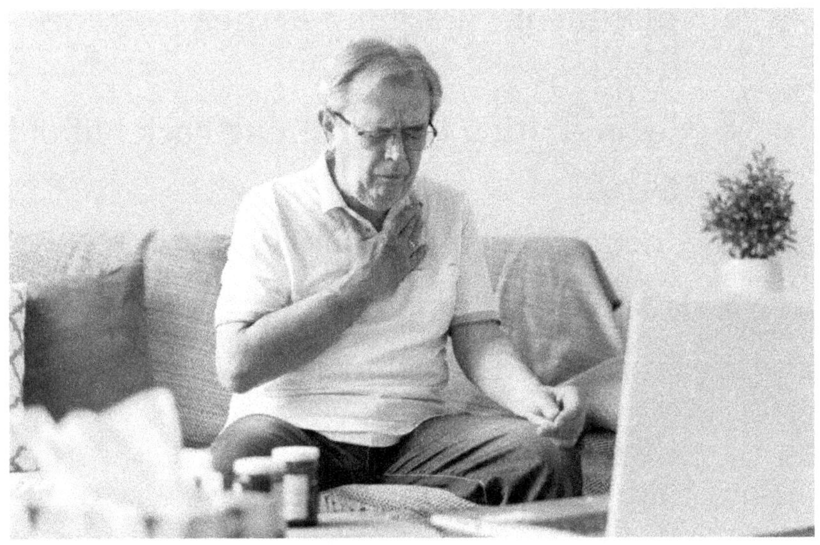

Sometimes, signs of dysphagia may not readily be apparent. Nevertheless, pay attention to the following warning signs or symptoms:

- Coughing or choking when eating or drinking
- Pain during swallowing
- Feeling like something is stuck in your throat

- Inability to swallow (in some cases, it might not be immediately apparent)

- Infrequent gurgling when eating or drinking

- Regurgitation (food coming back out of the body)

- Uncontrollable/random drooling

- Hoarse voice when talking

- Unexpected heartburn

- Unexplained weight loss

Note that this is not an exhaustive list of signs and symptoms. If something seems off, be sure to notify medical professionals immediately.

Complications and Implications

If you or someone you care about is in the process of recovering from a stroke, the healthcare team will conduct a thorough examination of the ability to swallow food and liquids. Depending on the assessment outcomes, they might involve a speech/language therapist or consult with an otolaryngologist (ENT doctor) to determine the next steps in the treatment regimen.

While the risk of dysphagia persists, even beyond the hospital environment, particularly if you choose home-based treatment or witness improvements in overall health during recovery, the likelihood of occurrence is minimal with consistent monitoring. If left unaddressed, the consequences can be severe, including the risk of choking or silent aspiration, potentially leading to complications like pneumonia. Timely intervention is crucial to prevent such complications and ensure a positive outcome in the recovery journey.

When is a Feeding Tube Needed?

In cases where dysphagia is severe and impedes the ability to swallow, the implementation of a feeding tube may be necessary. A percutaneous endoscopic gastrostomy (PEG) procedure is typically performed to insert the feeding tube, allowing direct delivery of nutrition to the stomach.

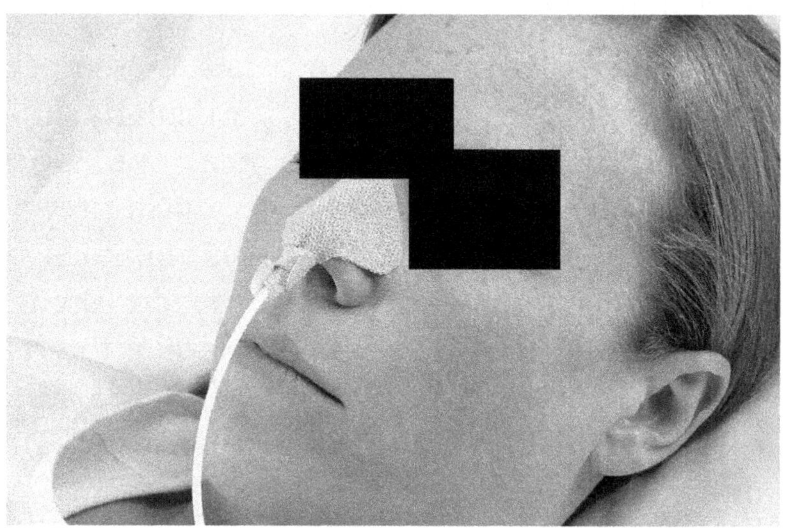

The PEG procedure involves the use of endoscopes, where small incisions are made to facilitate the insertion of tube-like devices into the body and the stomach to place the feeding tube. Local anesthesia is administered during the 20 to 30-minute procedure to ensure a painless experience. A dietitian will be available to provide guidance on the dietary aspects while using the feeding tube, also known as the G tube. Specialized nutrition and hydration will be administered through the G tube, which is approximately the size of a pen or pencil. It features an external bumper on one end to prevent further insertion into the stomach and a cap or plug on the other end to prevent leakage of stomach fluids onto the skin or clothes.

Throughout this period, doctors will offer advice on necessary precautions and signs to monitor, and it is crucial to communicate any complications experienced. Upon improvement of the condition, the tube can be removed, and the individual may eventually resume normal eating and drinking. Consultation with a doctor is recommended for guidance on post-removal procedures.

For elderly individuals and those dealing with dysphagia, adopting a soft diet may be recommended. Here are 10 easily swallowable recipes suitable for individuals with swallowing difficulties or dysphagia.

Nasogastric (NG) Feeding Tube

Alternatively, in certain situations, a nasogastric (NG) tube may be recommended. This tube is inserted through the nose, down the throat, and into the stomach. Typically employed for short-term feeding and administration of medications, NG tubes are commonly utilized for periods up to six weeks. Regular checks are necessary to ensure the stability of these tubes.

The placement of an NG tube can cause discomfort or mild pain, but the procedure is relatively brief and less invasive compared to the PEG process. Anesthetic lozenges may be provided to numb the upper gastrointestinal tract and alleviate any discomfort during the insertion process.

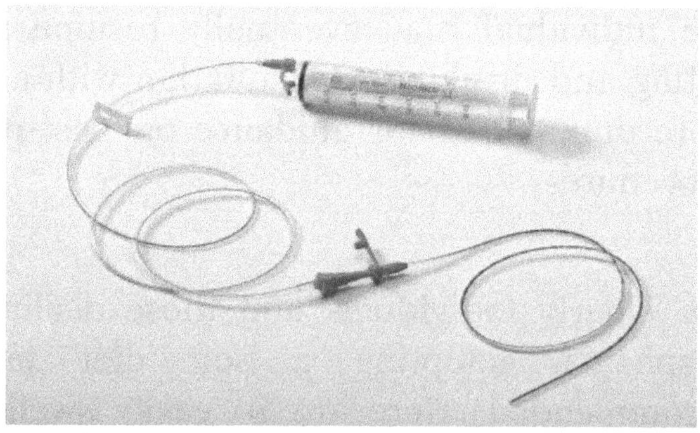

Who Treats Dysphagia?

A comprehensive and specialized team of medical professionals is typically essential for effective dysphagia treatment. Reiterating from earlier sections, these professionals play crucial roles:

- **Speech/Language/Swallowing Therapists:** These specialists assist in managing dysphagia, recommending therapies to restore the ability to swallow food and drink.

- **Dietitian:** Offers guidance on the recommended diet for the recovery process. In cases requiring a feeding tube, they provide advice on tube feeding.

- **Otolaryngologist (ENT Doctor):** Specialized in ear, nose, and throat-related complications.

- **Gastroenterologist:** Specializes in diagnosing and treating disorders of the digestive system.

- **Neurologist:** Consulted based on the stroke's severity to address lingering complications that may impact swallowing.

The Screening Process

Dysphagia screening involves a comprehensive assessment to evaluate the swallowing process and identify the location of dysphagia. Individuals may be required to swallow small amounts of different food types or water to assess their ability to swallow without issues. In some cases, swallowing solid food or a barium-coated pill may be necessary for X-ray observation, providing a clear view of movement for an accurate assessment.

Additional screening procedures that could be employed to determine the cause of dysphagia include:

- **Endoscopy:** Involves passing an endoscope down the throat to examine the condition of the esophagus and may include taking samples for further testing.

- **Fiber-optic Endoscopic Evaluation of Swallowing (FEES):** Similar to endoscopy, this procedure is designed to observe the swallowing process.

- **Imaging Scans:** CT or MRI scans may be conducted to generate detailed images of the throat and esophagus.

The **Dysphagia** Treatment Process

The treatment of dysphagia is determined by the type and cause of swallowing difficulties. In milder cases, learning exercises, such as specific swallowing techniques, may suffice to address the issue. This could involve acquiring skills like proper food placement in the mouth or adjusting body and head positions to facilitate swallowing. In some instances, significant modifications to eating habits may be necessary.

Other treatment approaches include:

- **Medications:** Prescribed to prevent acid reflux or manage esophageal spasms and other related issues.

- **Esophageal Dilation:** Involves using an endoscope with a specialized balloon to gently stretch the esophagus open. Alternatively, a flexible tube may be utilized instead of a balloon.

- **OnabotulinumtoxinA Injections:** This involves injecting a substance that relaxes the muscles at the end of the esophagus. Repeat injections may be necessary, and it may serve as a temporary solution.

- **Surgery:** Reserved for severe cases, followed by speech and swallowing therapy during the recovery process. Surgical procedures may involve making an incision to facilitate the passage of food and drink into the stomach.

Before undergoing any treatment, it's crucial to have a thorough discussion with the medical team. Prepare a list of questions to gain a comprehensive understanding of how the treatment will impact you, the expected outcomes, and other relevant details.

The Recovery Process

Dysphagia is typically a transient condition, and many individuals experiencing it will witness improvements over time. Stroke rehabilitation may be suggested to expedite the recovery process, aiding in the strengthening of swallowing muscles. This rehabilitation could involve learning techniques such as thoroughly chewing food before swallowing, adopting an upright posture while eating, and other beneficial practices, with guidance from a therapist.

Additionally, dietary modifications may be necessary, such as preparing soft or pureed foods to facilitate easier swallowing. A dietitian will provide recommendations on food and drink choices to ensure adequate nutritional intake, along with advising on items to be avoided to prevent complications. For instance, sticky foods might be eliminated from the diet due to their potential to complicate the swallowing process.

Here are additional measures you can take to aid in the recovery process:

- **Maintain oral hygiene:** Ensure good oral and dental health to prevent potential issues caused by bacteria in your mouth.

- **Eat and drink at a comfortable pace:** Avoid rushing the process, as doing so could lead to serious complications, such as food becoming lodged in your throat.

- **Refrain from eating or drinking when fatigued:** If you feel sleepy or weak, avoid consuming food or beverages to prevent the risk of items entering your windpipe.

- **Have someone present for support:** Having someone around can offer assistance with eating and drinking, as well as keep an eye on your well-being.

- **Seek clarification:** If you have any uncertainties or concerns, don't hesitate to communicate with your therapist or doctor for guidance.

Recovery will take some time, and it varies from person to person. Be sure to have someone by your side at all times, and don't hesitate to discuss your worries frankly with them. If need be, speak to a professional counselor to help you put your mind at ease. You don't have to do this alone.